Healthy Habits for Kids

By: Megan Austin

Healthy Habits for Kids
By: Megan Olivia Austin

Healthy Homestead Living
A division of Strive 4 Savvy, International S.A.
©2018 Strive 4 Savvy International S.A.
First Edition

Cover design done by Denise Barringer, Maddix Publishing
Typesetting, book layout, compilation, photography, and publishing done by Strive 4 Savvy, International. All photographs used in the book are either the property of Strive 4 Savvy, International, used with permission, or public domain.

Published by: Strive 4 Savvy, International & Maddix Publishing
Edited by: Strive 4 Savvy, International

ISBN: 978-1-7326471-2-1

Disclaimer: For educational and entertainment purposes only.
None of the information provided is intended to offer medical advice of any kind, nor is this this book intended to replace medical advice, nor to diagnose, prescribe, or treat any disease, condition, illness, or injury.

Author and publisher claim no responsibility to any person or entity for any liability, loss, or damage caused or alleged to be caused directly or indirectly as a result of the use, application, or interpretation of the material in this book.

Contents:

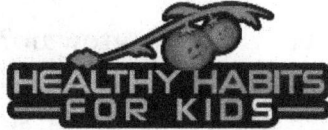

CHAPTER 1
What is a Habit?

What do you want to be when you grow up? An athlete? A doctor? Or maybe a teacher? Whatever you want to be, you have to be HEALTHY to do it well and be successful! Crazy right? No matter what you want to be when you grow up, it takes energy, mental toughness, thinking skills, and stamina to be successful.

Did you know that being healthy isn't just eating vegetables? It's true! Exercise, hygiene, and hydration are all important to being healthy. I'm not saying that if you don't exercise every day, or take a shower, or can't resist that cookie just that once, you're not healthy. I'm just saying, that it's important that you make good choices on a regular basis, because these all add up to create the overall condition of your health.

Hey, we all make mistakes once in awhile, and that's ok. When we make mistakes we learn. The goal is to make good choices MOST of the time so we can be healthy, energetic, feel good, do well, and HAVE FUN!

Oh, hold up! I forgot to introduce myself. My name is Megan, and I'm a kid just like you! Currently, I am 11 years old. I love playing computer games, swimming, riding bikes, and playing with my animals. Lucky for me, I was raised on a farm where we grow a lot of our own vegetables and fruits, and my parents have taught me healthy habits from an early age. As a result, I don't get sick very often (almost never), and I've never taken prescribed medicine from a doctor. So the stuff I'm sharing with you in this book really works!

What do I mean when I talk about the importance of "Healthy Habits"? Well, habits are things we do over and over, sometimes without even thinking about them. A habit can be good or bad. We want to set good habits, or *"Healthy Habits"*, as I like to call them, because they help us physically, mentally and spiritually. They can also help us become better siblings, better friends, better athletes, and better students. *Unhealthy Habits*, like eating too much sugar, staying up too late at night, or being lazy, can really be tempting. But, our Healthy Habits can conquer these unhealthy ones, if we choose to do them more often.

Don't worry, like I said, we all make mistakes sometimes and our mistakes can help us do better in the future. For example one cookie once in awhile won't kill you. We just don't want to have, like, 5 cookies a day…everyday!

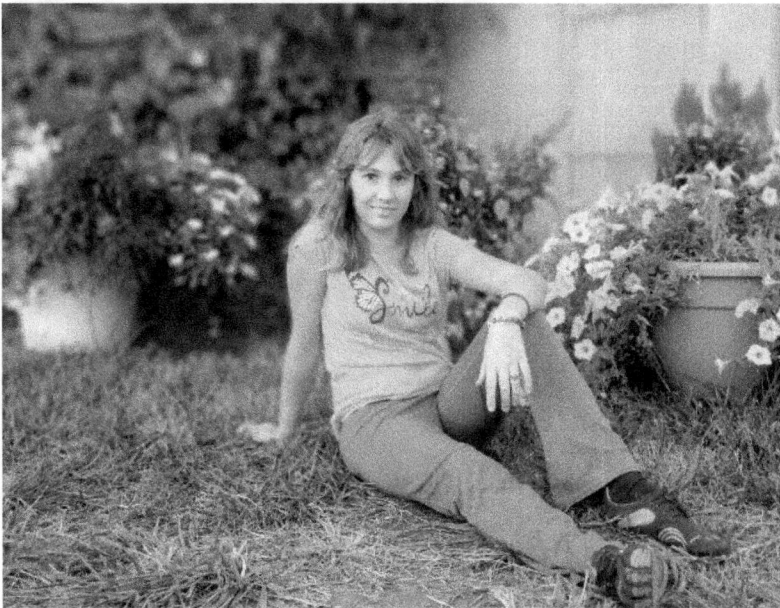

We want to get the into the habit of making smart choices as often as possible. Like I said, once in a while it's ok to have a cookie… or a whole box… (I've made that mistake before so don't feel bad), but I still try to eat healthy **most** of the time. Actually, you probably shouldn't do that; I don't advise eating a whole box of cookies at once. :/ They may taste good, but too many can make you sick.

Anyway, back to business.

Over time, I've developed habits that help me stay healthy. Habits that help me resist that temptation of sugar, for example. Ok, now I'm hungry. I think I want a nice big salad with tomatoes, cucumbers, carrots, and peas. Yep, delicious!

Oops, I'm getting side-tracked again. Back to habits. To me, habits are like goals that you accomplish every day. For instance, let's look at making your bed. Every day, let's say you have the goal of making your bed. After you do it everyday for a couple weeks, then it just comes naturally. Isn't it cool how your mind does that? Here's another example. If you have a pet, you have to take care of it. It may take some time, but sooner or later you get used to it and care for it every day. You don't have to think about it anymore like you did at first. Your parents don't have to remind you to feed your pet or take care of your pet, you just do it. The cool thing is, all habits are like this. The more you do them, the easier it gets. Some super- smart scientific adults say that it takes about 21 days

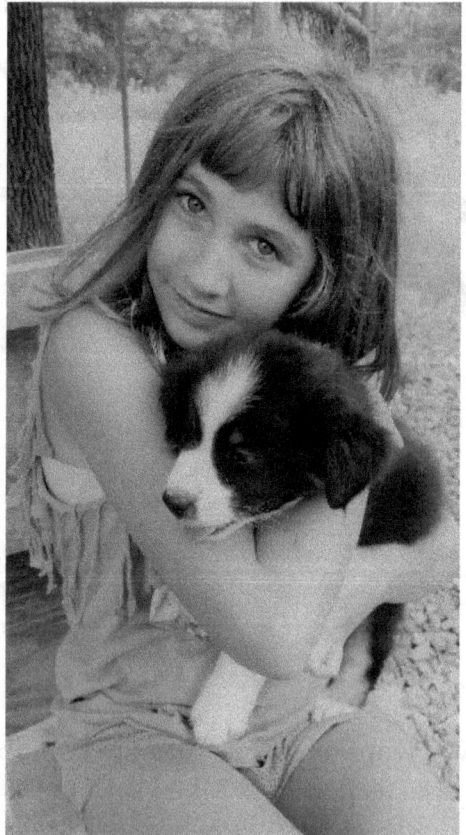

to turn an action into a habit. Is this true? Who knows? Whether it's 21 days or 51 days, repeating good choices over and over is always a good idea! Plus, developing healthy habits as kids, means there's a good chance we'll have healthy habits when we grow up. Cool, right?

Are you ready for my super awesome top Healthy Habits that I use to stay healthy, fit, and on top of my game? In the following chapters, I will share my favorites and show you why they can be great habits for you too!

CHAPTER 2

Habit 1:
Healthy Foods

Food. Everyone loves it. Food is very crucial to your body. Without it we would starve to death. We just want to make sure we eat the right food. Now, I bet you're asking yourself, "What is the *right* food?" Well, HEALTHY foods of course. Healthy foods, like fruits, vegetables, herbs and sprouts, are all amazing foods to eat.

Yeah, SPROUTS! I can't get enough of them! Once I start, it's hard for me to stop. Especially kale sprouts. (If you're not familiar with sprouts, they're basically baby plants, after the seeds start to grow. I highly recommend you try them.) Mmmmm! I think kale, broccoli, pea, or basil sprouts are the best! Anyway, a sprout is considered a superfood. What do I mean by superfood? Well, a superfood is generally something we eat that is very high in phytonutrients (fi-doh-noo-tree-ants). I know that seems like a long and confusing word, but it's a cool term for a substance found in plants, that is extremely good for your health. Those super smart scientists believe that phytonutrients are made when plants capture sunlight and convert it into energy.

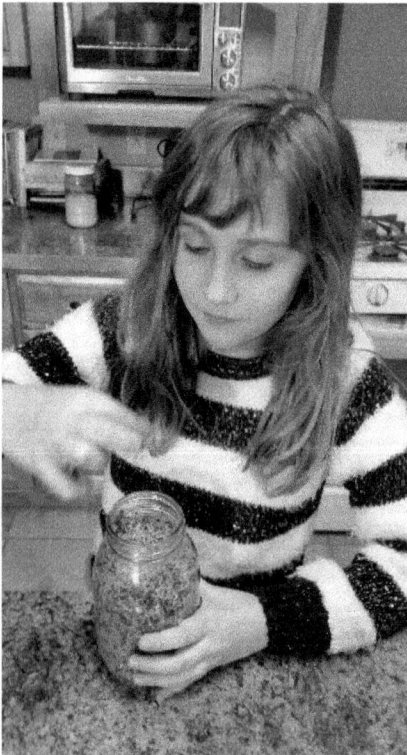

Did you know that superfoods aren't just vegetables and fruits? Yep! Some herbs, greens, oils, nuts, and seeds can be superfoods, too. And there are so many delicious superfoods to choose from, such as watermelon, strawberries, blueberries, avocado, and almonds.

Eating healthy means choosing foods that are good for us; foods that have things like vitamins, minerals, and other good stuff that feed our body and give us energy.

Plus, it means avoiding bad foods that can make us sick. Let's talk about a few of my favorite good foods and a few foods that you may not realize are unhealthy.

FRUITS AND VEGETABLES

Fruits and veggies are at the top of the list for good foods that are healthy. I'm often surprised by how many kids say they don't like vegetables. Do you like vegetables? No? Well have you tried HOME GROWN vegetables? Home grown foods always taste much better than store bought. Do you know why? First off, home grown vegetables are much more fresh. You can just pick something and eat it! (Once they're ready to be

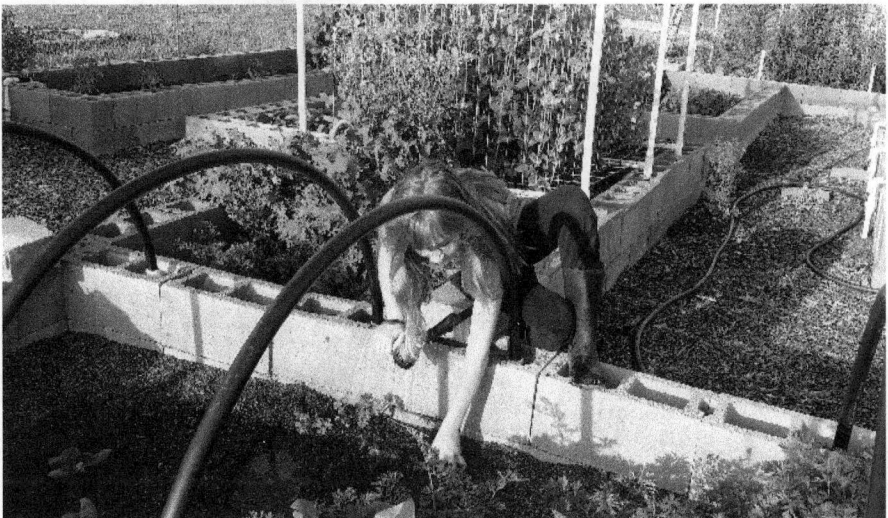

harvested). Also, did you know that many commercial farmers pick the vegetables before they're ripe? Some farmers will pick their crops so that they will last longer as they ship them to stores. For example, most tomatoes are picked green rather than red, because green tomatoes are more firm and don't bruise as easily when getting them from the farm to the store. Crazy, right?

I'm not saying that grocery store vegetables are bad. They're just not __as__ good as home grown. Plus, home grown foods taste way better. If you don't think you like vegetables now, then maybe you should try REAL, FRESH vegetables. Put that delicious healthy plant in your mouth and your taste buds are going to have a party! Woo hoo! Lots of times I have friends or other kids visit our homestead who get to eat fresh vegetables from the garden, sometimes for the first time, and they always enjoy them. Even kids who say they normally don't eat vegetables. Peas, carrots, tomatoes, lettuce,…. As they say, don't knock it until you try it!

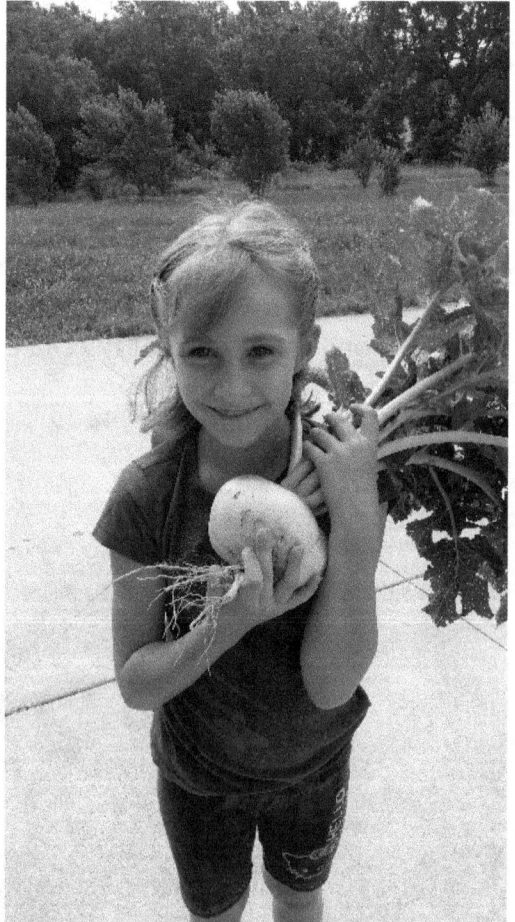

If you don't have access to home-grown, that's ok too. No matter where they come from or how they are grown, fruits and vegetables are some of the best things you can eat. You can get more fresh veggies at organic stores and occasionally a farmer's market, too. The price isn't always higher either. The goal is to get the freshest, ripest, varieties, because that's where the best flavor comes from (and the most nutrients).

Still don't think you like vegetables? Did you know that fruits and vegetables come in multiple varieties and colors? If you don't think you like vegetables, maybe you just haven't found the right *kinds* yet. For example, carrots aren't always just orange. Have you ever tried a purple carrot? What? *Purple* carrots? Yep. And carrots can be yellow, red, or white too! Personally, I think purple carrots taste even better than orange ones. Tomatoes can be red, but they can also be orange, yellow, green, purple, white, striped, and speckled! Just about any fruit or vegetable comes in different colors, sizes, flavors, and varieties. So, if you don't like one kind, maybe you'll like a different kind instead.

Still don't think you like vegetables? Try cooking them differently. Flavors change quite a bit depending on how they are prepared.

For example, I'm not a big fan of canned peas, but I love them fresh or steamed. I like broccoli too, but I think it's much better steamed or raw. My mom loves broccoli roasted, but that's not my favorite way to eat them. Think of it as an adventure, and explore which are your favorite kinds and how you like them cooked. You may find out that you DO like vegetables after all!

MEAT

Just like fruits and vegetables, meat can be important too. Not everyone eats meat, and that's ok. If you do eat meat, you have to be careful which meats you eat, though. Processed meat, pork, shrimp, and crab are all examples of meats that can be unhealthy, especially processed meat like hot dogs, sandwich meat, and chicken nuggets… all things that many of my friends say they eat all the time.

Now I bet you are asking yourself, "WHAAAAAAAT?????
PORK???? THAT MEANS BACON IS UNHEALTHY?!!!!!!!!
Chicken nuggets, too? Why?"

Great question! There is a very logical explanation to why pork
and some other meats are considered less healthy. And
remember, I'm not saying you can NEVER eat these things. Just
make better choices more regularly. And, there are great healthy
alternatives out there too, that taste great! (Like turkey bacon.)

Have you ever really thought about where meat comes from?
Meat is basically the muscle from different animals. Pork, like
bacon, ham, and sausage, comes from pigs. Pigs will eat pretty
much anything that can fit in their mouths, including the bad
stuff. After the animal consumes their "*food*", the toxins from
what they have eaten get into their bloodstream, which then
finds its way into their muscle, and that's what we eat.

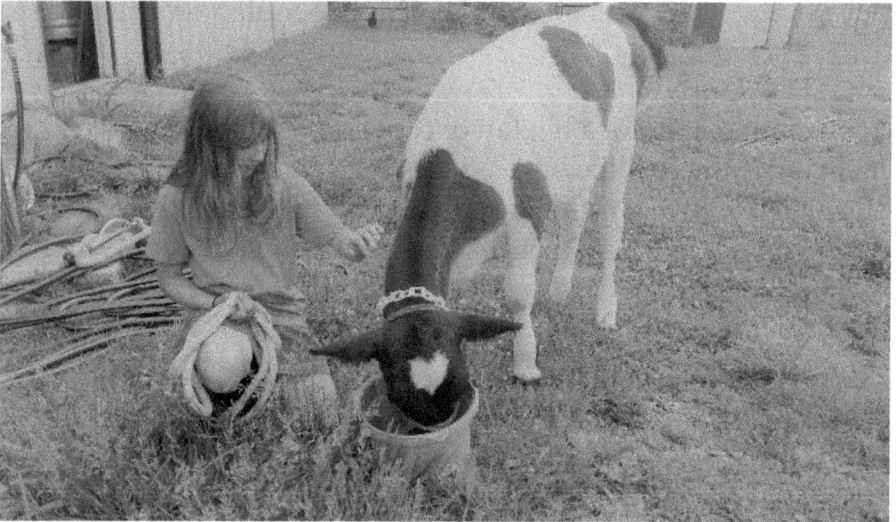

Therefore, we consume the toxins in the meat. These toxins can
make it harder for our bodies to be healthy. And like I said, it's
not just pork. Processed meats are like that too? Yep. Processed
meats are those that have been mixed with other ingredients and
processed in some way, like heating, curing, or pressing. They

may taste good, but they have lots of yucky, unhealthy ingredients added to them. (To me they don't taste very good, either). Some of these ingredients can make it harder for your body to function. So even though they may make your tongue happy, they don't make the rest of your body very happy.

The best meats to eat are the ones that come from healthy, organic animals and haven't been processed. Some of my favorites are chicken, turkey (good any time, not just Thanksgiving), salmon, cod, steak, and hamburger.

SUGARS

I love sugar. I have a really big sweet tooth. Sugar is found almost everywhere. Energy drinks, sodas, donuts, candy, canned foods like sweetened applesauce, processed foods, and even things like toothpaste, have sugar in them. I love sugar just as much as anyone, but too much can be a problem.

Do you know what sugar does to you? First off, it can make you tired so you won't want to do anything. This is because when you swallow sugar or something with a large enough amount of sugar, your blood sugar level increases, giving you a large burst of energy, that at first may seem like a good thing, but after a while though, the storm passes by, and you start to feel tired while the body tries to re-balance its blood sugar. Some people call it a "Sugar Crash."

The most unhealthy sugar is refined white sugar. Once consumed, the sugar goes right into your bloodstream. That sugar feeds bad bacteria which can then grow and form infections. Hmm. That reminds me of a story.

My mom is an expert in health and nutrition. A few years ago, my dad got cancer. As part of his treatment, we went on a special diet to help him heal. This diet eliminated all forms of sugar, but guess what? We still could have "sweets". Instead of eating sugar, we used an herb called stevia. Stevia is healthy and still very sweet, and unlike regular sugar, it doesn't feed the bad bacteria or affect blood sugar levels! And guess what? Even with no sugar, we still made brownies, cookies, and even sweetened our tea with stevia. Cool right?

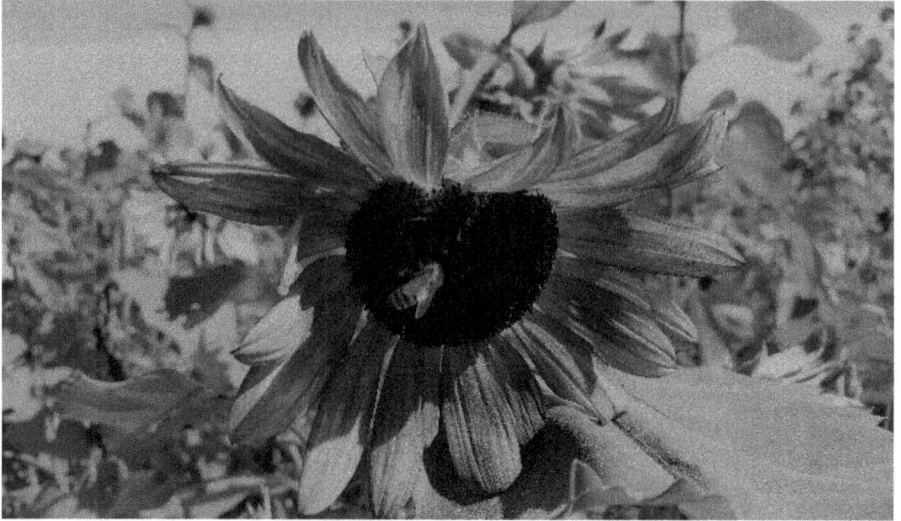

Another healthy sweetener is honey. Honey is made by honeybees, and not only tastes super good, but has nutrients in it that can help with health. So even if you have a sweet tooth like me, you can still enjoy treats while sticking with this important healthy habit of healthy eating. Don't forget, fruits make great healthy "sweet" treats, too. Healthy "sweets" like fruit, honey and stevia taste AMAZING! I definitely recommend them.

FAST FOODS

Everyone loves some kind of fast food. I mean, who doesn't? But fast foods are often very unhealthy. You can tell by the taste of most fast food and whole foods, which is which. If you eat a chicken nugget from the drive-thru, and a chicken from a homestead, the chicken from the homestead probably tastes better. Like 10,874 times better.

Also, do you know how that chicken nugget was made? Well for starters it came from a chicken, (obviously). But then it was processed, usually with added sugar or it's evil health-stealing friend, High Fructose Corn Syrup. Both are very unhealthy.

Second, have you ever read the ingredients on a label of processed food? Most of the time you don't even know what some of those words mean or how to pronounce them! That's because they're usually chemicals made in a lab.

Yeah, fast food may taste good, but boy is it unhealthy. Plus, I'd rather have homemade ice cream with stevia and one of my dad's grilled hamburgers and my mom's special potato fries, than those same foods from any fast food place. There's just no comparison!

SALT

I love salt. It adds just the perfect touch to a lot of foods we eat. Some of which are potatoes, pretzels, and chips. Can you

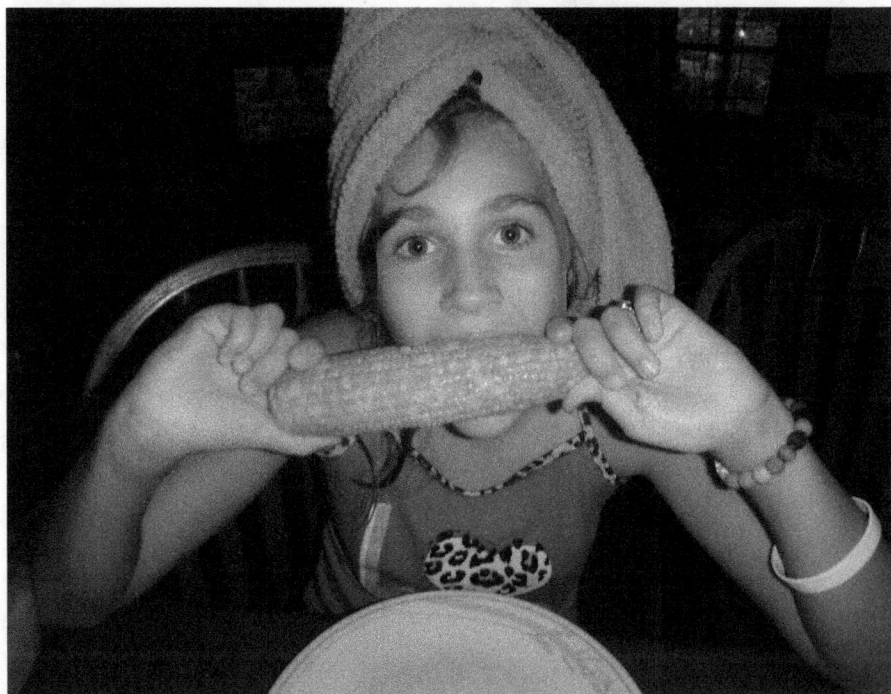

imagine eggs without salt? Or sweet corn without salt? Salt is also used for baking. But there are different kinds of salt, and some are healthy…and some are actually very bad for you. So, what salt do you use?

Lots of people use table salt, most commonly being refined white salt. Salt is a combination of two minerals: sodium and chloride. Your body needs all sorts of minerals, like Iron, Magnesium, and others, but we're going to focus on salt, which is mostly sodium and chloride.

Have you ever asked yourself "Where did this food come from?" Well I can tell you where the salt came from. Most table salts come from underground. Yep! Then, in the case of refined white salt, which is what most people think of when I talk about salt, the salt gets processed, taking away the good healthy stuff like other minerals, and giving the salt that white color.

Did you know that there is such a thing as PINK salt? Well there is, and it's very healthy too. It's called Himalayan salt. Another healthy salt is called Celtic Sea Salt. That's the one my family uses. Himalayan Pink salt and Celtic Sea salt are not processed or refined and still have all the good stuff still in them. Plus, they taste better!

Do you ever feel thirsty after consuming salt? I do sometimes. But did you know that you need salt to stay hydrated? Yep! It's important to have a balance between salt, water, and other minerals. That's why sometimes you crave salty foods.

Sometimes your body needs more of the minerals found in salt. Using healthy salts can actually help your body stay hydrated and give your body important minerals. What do I mean by staying hydrated? Read on to Chapter 3 to find out!

CHAPTER 3
Habit 2: Hydration

Wait a minute,… all this talk about healthy foods… but we're missing something,… but what? A drink, that's what we're missing! Something tasty to wash down the delicious, HEALTHY food. Hmm… What should I have? Sweet tea? No… Soda? No… Oh! I know! How about a large glass of WATER? Soooo refreshing! <Slurp> Now that I think about it, I made the right choice by drinking water. But why?

For starters, do you know how much sugar is in soda? One can of Sprite has 33 grams of sugar, Coke has 39 grams, and Mountain Dew has 77 grams! It's still ok to have a little bit of soda once in awhile, but just imagine if that's all you drank! I'm sure that I would be SO tired, I wouldn't be able do do anything but sleep! (Remember what I said earlier about the sugar crash?)

Guess how much sugar is in water? Just take a guess. Five grams? Three grams? Oh come on! It has to be one. But no, it's ZERO. There is NO SUGAR in pure water. None, zero, zilch. And that's PURE WATER; no artificial flavors. But you can add your own flavors by soaking fruits, herbs, or cucumbers in the water. I like to do that.

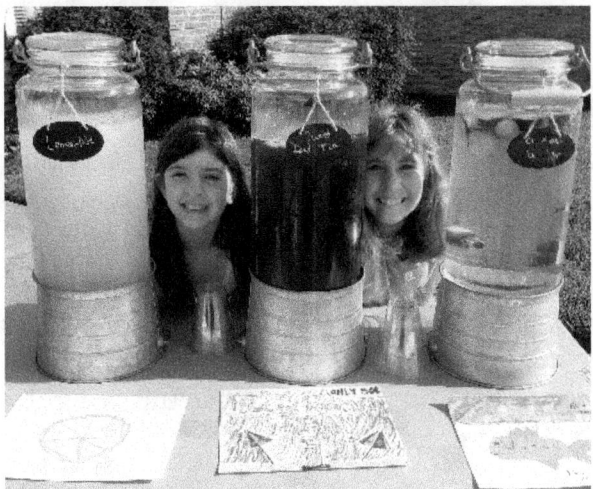

Why is water the best?

Ok, this is probably a really easy question to answer. The answer is clear (Like water. Get it?). Water is healthy. But what if someone asked you, *"why?"* Again, really easy answer; water has no sugar. Yes, that is true. But is that the only reason why water is healthy? Nope!

The human body is made up of about 70% water. Without water you become dehydrated. Like I said in the salt section, the body needs hydration to function. Without it, the cells *"deflate."* Your cells, blood, organs, and even brain, all need water to function!

Here's a great tip on making sure you drink enough water each day. Drink a big glass of water with lemon when you first wake up in the morning. Drinking water when you wake up helps get your body going. The lemon makes it taste good, but also helps your body to stay hydrated and balanced. Plus, the lemon helps you wake up after sleeping for so long. Then, the rest of the day, carry a water bottle so that you have fresh water with you wherever you are and whatever you are doing. That way you can keep sipping throughout the day.

How much water should I drink per day?

The amount of water you should drink per day depends on your body weight. You should drink at least half your body weight in ounces per day. So if you weigh 80 pounds, you would have to drink at least 40 ounces. That's about five average glasses. But let's say you had P.E. class today, and you ran seven laps around the gym. You feel thirsty right? That's because sometimes, like when you do exercise or when it's hot outside, you need even more water. So start with half your weight, and increase if you are sweating or if it's a hot day.

Did you know, there are multiple ways that water exit's your body? Some of those are when you sweat, cry, and even when you breathe. That's why if your crying, you usually feel better after taking a drink of water. Super cool right? Part of the reason why you need to drink at least half your bodyweight in water is because you lose so much of it. It's important to regain the water that you naturally lose on a daily basis.

Other healthy drinks that you can also enjoy sometimes (as long as you mostly drink water) include herbal tea, kombucha, nut milks, and smoothies.

Fruit juices turn to sugar in our bodies so be careful how often your drink them. Even though I love them and they taste really good, it's best if they are more like a dessert or treat than a drink.

All this talk about water is making me thirsty. Time to get a big drink of cool, refreshing water! <Slurp!> Ahh!

CHAPTER 4
Habit 3: Get Up and GO!!!!

Do you ever feel tired and lazy? There are plenty of reasons why you could be tired. Some of those reasons are lack of exercise, not enough sleep, a poor diet, and a negative mental mindset (more on that later). Your body naturally needs movement for physical and mental fitness. In some cases, just fidgeting with your pencil a bit can help. Some super smart scientific-type grown ups have figured out that some kids learn and remember better while moving or fidgeting. These scientists say movement while learning is especially helpful to most boys. For example, my dad likes to pace when he's on the phone. I know a couple kids who prefer to stand instead of sit at their desks sometimes at school. Just remember to not let fidgeting distract you from your tasks or from your assignments at school. ;)

Exercise is an important Healthy Habit. But when I say exercise, I mean doing something that involves movement and increasing your heart rate. This can be anything, and it should always be fun. Remember when I said the more you do your habits every day the easier it gets? It's like that with exercising too! The more you exercise, the easier it gets.

It's ok to push yourself just a little too. I mean how else would you get better? All I'm saying, is exercise at least 30 minutes to an hour a day. Now, this doesn't have to be lifting weights. You could be exercising by running, doing jumping jacks and push ups, or even swimming, bouncing on a trampoline, or just walking. Whatever you do, do it every day.

If you're just sitting around playing video games and not getting the physical exercise you need, you may begin to feel tired and lazy. Now, this may not be the case for you. Maybe you already get enough exercise. If that's you, awesome! Still, you may want to keep reading this chapter just in case you want to get some new ideas or share it with your friends.

HOW MUCH EXERCISE SHOULD I GET IN A DAY?

Some may say you need 30 minutes a day, and some may say you need 45 minutes. Ages six and up, need at least one hour of exercise every day, according to some experts. Sound like a lot? It really isn't. When you think about it, there's a whole 24 hours in a day. So what's spending just one of those hours doing some fun movement to help you stay fit? For most Elementary kids, recess and sports cover lots of that hour. Options at home could be running, jumping jacks, push ups, shooting hoops, riding your bike, or just about anything where your heart gets beating a little faster... Now, maybe you're in Middle School and don't have recess. But even if that's you, there is still plenty of time left

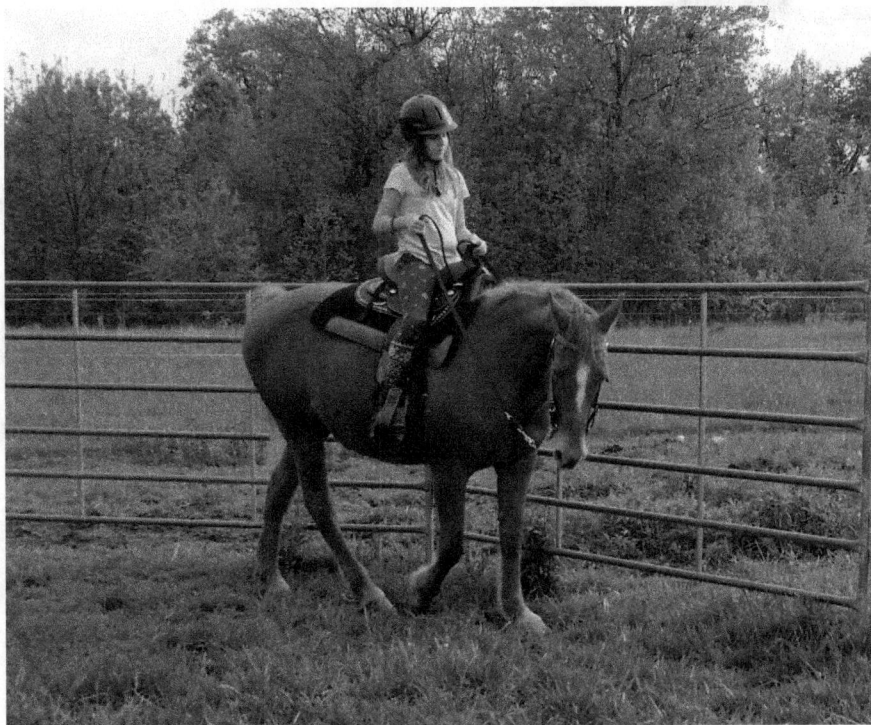

in the day for some activities that get you moving. What are your favorites?

Make it fun!!!!

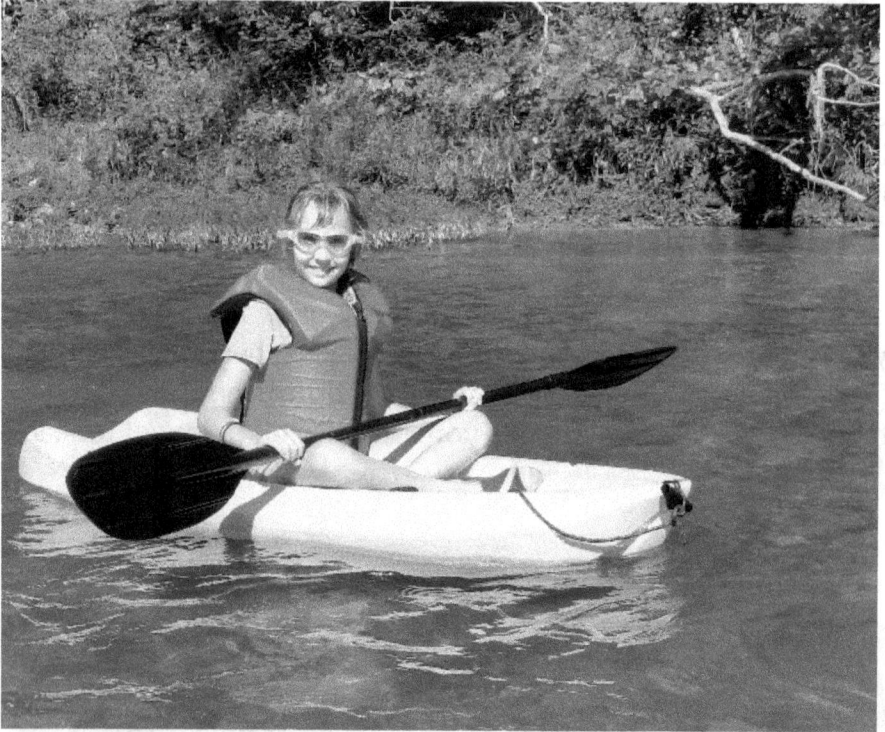

Hey! Exercise doesn't have to be work. You're a kid!!!!! And as a kid, we're all about fun, right? Why not play some music? You could just dance as your exercise. It's better than just playing on electronics all day. I know I repeat that a lot, but it's true. I love my electronics, too, but as my mom often says, it's all about balance.

I hate doing stuff that's not fun. I mean, who would want to? But sometimes we can MAKE things fun. So what's fun to you? Do you like watching TV? Watch a movie while doing your push ups or walking on a treadmill. Do you like eating? Reward yourself with a healthy snack like an apple or a carrot when you're done with your exercise. NO SUGAR! Remember the cookie! Have a pet? Take them for a walk. Don't have a pet? Offer to walk a neighbor's dog. Dogs make great company, too. I don't advise walking a cat, though. They're not really the best at paying attention. If you live in a suburban area, why not ride a bike or run over to your friend's house? There are tons of fun things you can do to get some good exercise in each day!

What and what not to do while exercising

We want to have fun exercising, but there are some things that we want to avoid doing. Being safe is the number one priority.

First, you want to stretch. If you're running, this is really important. You can get muscle cramps very easily. Recently, we had Track and Field Fun Day at my school. I didn't have time to stretch, so I got a small cramp in my leg. Your muscles need to warm up before strenuous activity. Before running and jumping, I definitely want to stretch! Some ways you can stretch are by touching your toes, doing the butterfly, or the "W" stretch. That's where you sit down, spread your legs, and reach as far as you can down the center. There are many other stretches too. Stretches aren't just for the lower part of your body. You can stretch your arms, your neck, and your back too. One fun way to stretch is by doing yoga. Yoga not only stretches your muscles, but it helps with stress and makes you stronger!

The second thing you want to avoid when exercising is drinking or eating too much before exercising. You still may want to drink a little bit before exercising for hydration, but don't drink too much. This can cause muscle cramps as well. This caution is especially important if you are going swimming. That's why adults usually say to wait at least 30 minutes after eating before going swimming. You don't want to get a muscle cramp when you are in the water!

Just remember, don't hesitate to drink all the water you want after your exercising!!!!! Drinking water is one of the healthiest habits, and it makes you feel good! If you're really hot and thirsty, don't drink milk or energy drinks. Once in a while it's ok to have some, but not when you need to cool off from exercising. On really hot days when you're really sweaty, you can add some lemon, cucumber, mint, or strawberries to your water. That makes it taste good and gives you extra cooling nutrients.

Whatever exercise you choose, just make sure you do it every day and HAVE FUN!

Chapter 5

Habit 4: Wash up!

What is Hygiene, and why is it important?

Hygiene is a funny word that means keeping clean. This means taking a shower or bath every day and using soap. This also means washing your hair and brushing your teeth. For our older friends, make sure you keep a deodorant close by, though I'm sure you already do. No one wants to stink!

Hygiene is very important. Not to gross you out, but did you know, that tiny microscopic creatures are living on your body? They won't hurt you. They're called bacteria. Sometimes we just call them "germs". We have bacteria inside our bodies and outside our bodies. But some bacteria is good and some is bad. The "bad" germs are the ones that make us sick and also the ones that make us smell bad. We want to wash the bad germs out and keep the good ones. This helps us stay healthy.

If you don't wash regularly, you'll probably give off a bad body odor, which means you smell bad. And we don't want that, now do we? Taking a bath or shower helps our bodies get rid of the bad germs that make us smell. We should take a bath or shower every day...and if you go outside and get all hot and sweaty you may need to take a shower more than once in a day! If you are in a position where you can't take a shower, you can always wash up with a washcloth and use deodorant.

Did you know that your skin is the largest organ in your body? Your skin is actually one of the ways your body gets rid of toxins (the bad stuff inside your body from the things you eat and the chemicals you are exposed to). Sweating is one way your body naturally cools itself, but it is also one way your body cleans the inside. Stinky sweat is one indication that you have lots of toxins your body is trying to get rid of! The healthier you eat and live, the less stinky your sweat.

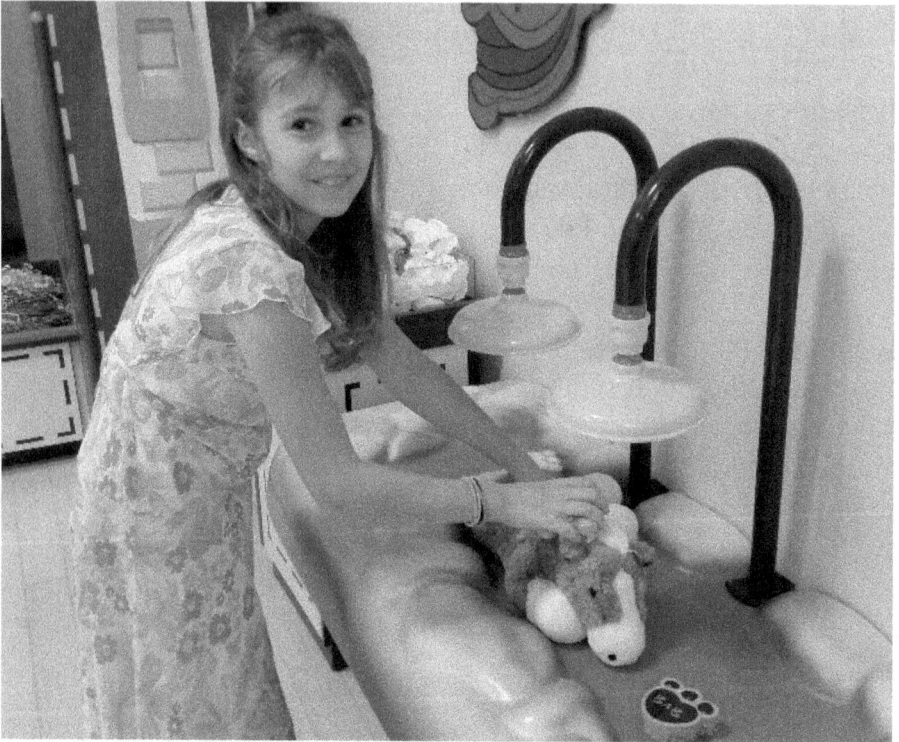

It's crazy how many kids don't like taking baths or showers. If you don't like taking showers, I don't know what to tell you other than maybe ask you why. Maybe try using a really fun soap that you really love the smell of, or put some music on to sing to while you are in the shower. Add some sudsy bubbles to the bath or some essential oils. Just be sure to be really thorough when you clean and get your whole body. Don't forget between your toes!

Dental Hygiene

Part of hygiene and taking care of yourself is keeping your teeth clean too. This means brushing your teeth every morning after breakfast and every night before bed. Brushing and flossing are important in keeping your teeth clean. So, why do we want to keep our teeth clean? Well, once we lose our baby teeth and get our adult teeth, these are the only teeth we get! We can't grow new ones if the ones we have go bad.

If we don't take care of our teeth, we can get cavities. Cavities can do serious damage to your teeth, which I'm sure you already know. But did you also know that cavities come from bad bacteria in your mouth? Bad bacteria comes in many forms, and most of the bad bacteria loves to feed on sugar. Makes sense, right? So when you eat foods with sugar, bacteria in your mouth also feed on the sugar. Then, the bad bacteria give off a waste product which is very acidic. That substance is what creates the holes in people's teeth. Pretty gross, right?

Flossing is also important. If you don't floss, stuff can build up in places your brush can't reach. Sometimes this can lead to painful teeth or teeth loss.

I recently visited my dentist for a check up (always a good idea, and dentists are cool ...not scary at all!). My dentist said a few things that I thought were pretty interesting.

One, was that a part of taking care of your teeth is eating the right foods. Hmm, where have we heard this before? :-) So, I bet you are wondering, "What does eating the right foods have to do with my teeth?" Well, food has to enter your body somehow right? Where does that food have to go before it's digested? That's right, your mouth. The sugar in unhealthy food can , as you know, create cavities, but the nutrients in the healthy food can help your teeth be stronger, add to the good bacteria in your mouth, and fight off the bad bacteria that is trying to live there.

My dentist also said that some drinks are really bad for your teeth. Because of the amount of sugar in them, some drinks that can be bad for your teeth are soda, sports drinks, and apple juice.

The other thing that I thought was interesting that my dentist told me was that healthy teeth also need saliva. The spit in your mouth actually helps protect your teeth from cavities. So if your mouth gets dry too much, you could be at a higher risk for teeth problems. My dentist recommended drinking lots of water (hmmm, where have we heard that before?) and chewing sugar-free gum. Occasionally chewing gum can actually make your body produce more saliva, and the gum can sometimes help clean your teeth. Just make sure it's sugar-free!

So be sure to brush, floss, drink lots of water, avoid too much sugar (especially in drinks), and enjoy chewing sugar-free gum. Those healthy habits will make your teeth smile. Plus, it's much more fun when you go to the dentist and the doctor says "Your teeth look great!," rather than "Ummmmm, you need to brush your teeth better."

Hair

Taking care of your hair is just as important as taking care of everything else. If you don't wash your hair, you have a higher risk of scalp infections and other health problems.

How many times a week do you wash your hair? Most kids my age (11) would wash their hair almost every other day, washing after getting in the pool as well. If you're younger than me, I suggest washing 3 to 4 times

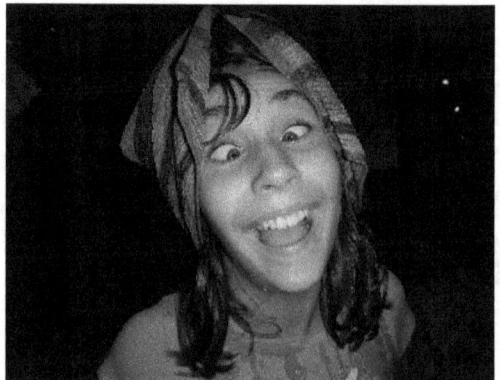

a week, and whenever your hair gets dirty.

Don't forget to brush your hair regularly, too. Brushing your hair can help get rid of all those icky dead skin cells. And brushing your hair can make it nice and pretty too without all those annoying tangles. The longer your hair, the more often you may need to brush.

Oh! One more thing. If you look clean, smell clean, and feel clean, you'll notice you have more confidence. You feel more like trying your best! We all love knowing we look good and being clean is a very important part of that.

Environment

Keeping your environment clean is also a good idea, particularly your bedroom. Your bedroom is your place... Your place to have fun, be creative, and get away from everything else. My mom calls my bedroom my "sanctuary". My place to be me, to be creative, or to relax.

It's a little harder to enjoy if your room is messy. Here are a few tips to keeping your room clean:

- Making your bed in the morning can freshen up your room. Create a habit of making your bed first thing every morning.
- If you have a lot of trash in your room, keep a trash can near by and empty it regularly.
- You might want to have a lot of shelves and baskets for toys and books. Stay organized as much as possible.
- Have a laundry hamper, so there's not a lot of dirty cloths just laying around.
- If you share a room with someone else, you can at least do your part, and also show this book to your

roommate if they can't keep their part of the room clean.

If you keep your room clean, coming home from school and relaxing on your made bed, can be much more refreshing.

So as you can see, creating healthy habits of keeping your body, teeth, hair, and room clean will help you in many ways.

One last thing we haven't talked about that you want to make an effort to keep "clean", and that is your MIND. I'll share more what I mean, later in this book… stay tuned!

Chapter 6

Habit 5: Sweet dreamZ Z z z z zz

Why is sleep important?

Sleep is really important for health, which is why I include it as another healthy habit. When we were babies, we slept all the time. As we got older, we slept a little less, but still took naps. Depending on how old you are now, you may not take naps anymore and just sleep at night, and sometimes you may stay up really late. If you were to stay up late every night, and wake up at 6 a.m. in the morning to get ready for school, you may start to regret it. Why? When you sleep, your mind is at rest, and that's when your body heals. Sleep is also when your body grows and develops, and as a kid that's really important. Usually you want to get 8 to 12 hours of sleep per night. If you don't get enough sleep over and over again, it can show in your face, attention span, and energy level. Getting enough sleep helps with your health, energy, concentration, and many other things. Make it a healthy habit to get a good night's sleep every night. I'm not saying that once in awhile you can't stay up late. I do that when I go to my Grandma's house! It's fun to stay up late from time to time for special occasions. You just wouldn't want to do it too often!

Tips on how to get a good night's sleep

We don't want to just sleep, we want to sleep well. Here are a few tips on how to sleep well:

- Turn off technology at least an hour before bed. This can give your eyes a break from the screen, and let your mind settle down. I know this is a tough one for me. It's just sooooo much fun. My mom's always telling me to turn

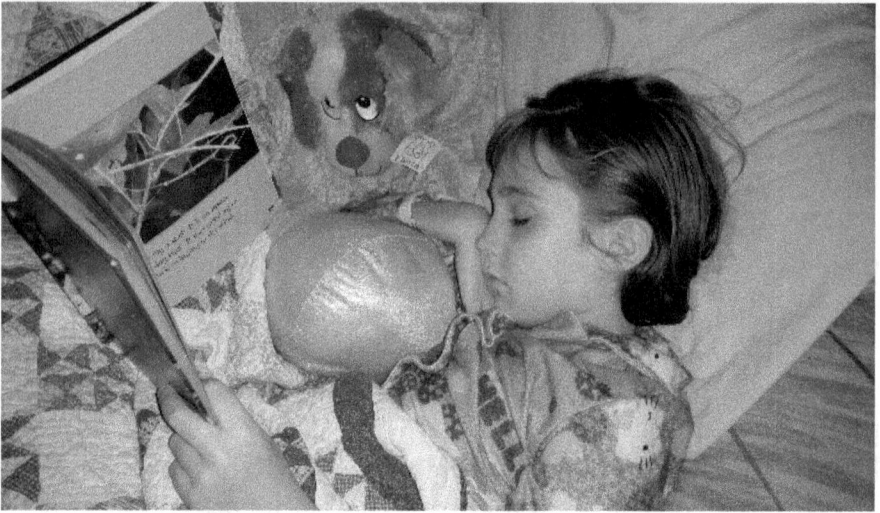

the technology off. Did you know that technology usually has a certain kind of blue light that tells your brain to stay awake? It's true! So turning off the phone, TV, or computer at least a couple hours before bed will help tell your brain it's time to sleep.

- Don't watch scary movies before bed. Some people can have bad dreams after watching a scary movie before bed.

- No sugar or caffeine before bed. This can keep you awake.

- Maybe have some magnesium before bed. This can help you relax. You can find it at most health food stores.

- Don't eat right before bed. You body needs time to digest. When you're sleeping your body gets confused. Is it time to rest??? Or is it time to digest??? My mom says we should avoid eating at least two hours before bedtime. Sometimes I get a little hungry before bed and need a small snack. In those cases, we stick with a green juice, a little bit of almond butter, or some soup. That way the snack doesn't mess with the body trying to sleep.

- Essential oils can really help with sleep. Using the right ones, like lavender and roman chamomile, can really give you a good night sleep. I use essential oils a lot before bed, and include them in my everyday life.

- Be comfortable! Make sure you have the right pillow, the room is the right temperature, and if you need a night light, use one, but your body tends to sleep better in the dark. Maybe have your favorite stuffed animal with you. I have this dog stuffed animal, that I've slept with ever since I was 4. His name is Rover...

- If you have a phone, don't plug it in next to your bed. Those super smart scientist people found out recently that having technology too close to your head when you sleep can actually affect your body in many negative ways, including poor sleep quality, difficulty concentrating, and getting sick more often. Plug in your phone, tablet, computer, etc. somewhere away from your bed. It's even better if it's in a completely different room!

So, as you can see, creating the healthy habit of sleep at an early age, helps your mind, your body, and your spirit, and will benefit you even as you become a grown up. Lots of adults have trouble sleeping, so setting up this important healthy habit now will help you a long time and avoid problems later.

Chapter 7

Habit 6: Mental Toughness

What is mental toughness?

Mental toughness is not your physical health, but your metal health, meaning your mindset, and how you react to different circumstances. It means how healthy you are internally. Remember what I said about keeping your mind "clean"? Let's look at a few areas of mental toughness healthy habits.

Confidence

Having a lot of confidence at an early age, can really affect you in a positive way during adulthood. For some kids, confidence can be a bit of a struggle. I know, because it still is sometimes for me too. And that's ok. Remember, we're all learning. If that's you, here are a few tips on gaining confidence that I use to continually grow in confidence:

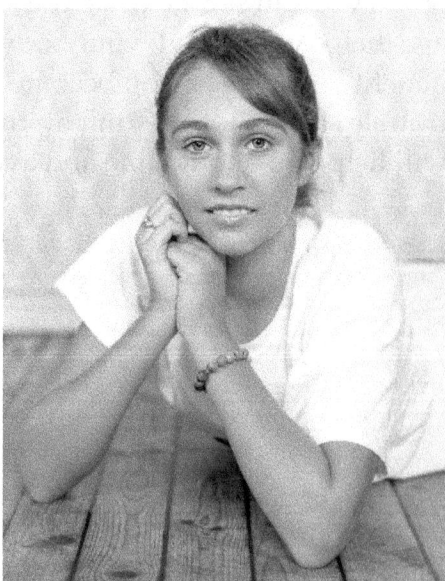

- If your parents will let you, when you go to restaurants, order for yourself instead of telling your mom or dad to tell the waiter or waitress. I remember doing that for the first time. Me, my dad, and my mom went to a restaurant, and I ordered for myself while my parents ordered for themselves. It was a great feeling to be able to speak for myself, even in such a simple way.

- Positive self talk is a big one. Some kids say bad things about themselves, because of their environment, and their peers. My chiropractor says to give myself 30 compliments every day even if I don't think they're true. It's actually a fun exercise. One way to keep track is to say one complement for every letter of the alphabet, and just come up with 4 more. For example: I am Awesome! I am Beautiful! I am Creative! …. You get the picture. My mom and I have fun doing this together. Some letters (like Q and X can take some creativity, but that makes it all the more fun.) If you catch yourself saying something bad about yourself, change it up and give yourself more compliments.

- Focus on gratitude. Be grateful for what you have. It's ok to want more, but be grateful that you have a shelter, food and clean water. Feeling grateful shifts your focus to the positive. No matter what your situation, there are always things you can feel grateful for. Some people recommend keeping a gratitude journal. This is actually fun and gives you something to look back on when you are having days that are particularly tough.

- Teamwork! Like they say, "teamwork makes the dreamwork!" When you work together as a team on something, you support each other, work towards a common goal, and help build each other up. If you like sports, being a part of a sports team works, but if you aren't really into sports, other types of teams work too!

So now, use these awesome confidence tips, and use them in your daily life. Don't forget to encourage others to do the same!

Help others

Helping others can feel good, knowing you made someone else's day. Even the most simple action can make a difference. But how about helping your parents? Why not just take like 15 minutes and do some extra chores? I'll bet they'll like that! It also feels good when you're done!

How about giving back? Let's say you want this really, really cool toy that your friend has, and they decide to give it to you. What do you do now? Other than being polite and telling them how much you appreciate them? Maybe they want this super cool toy you have?

Instead of just thinking about yourself, you could give the toy they like to your friend. Now that was just one example. There are many ways you could give back.

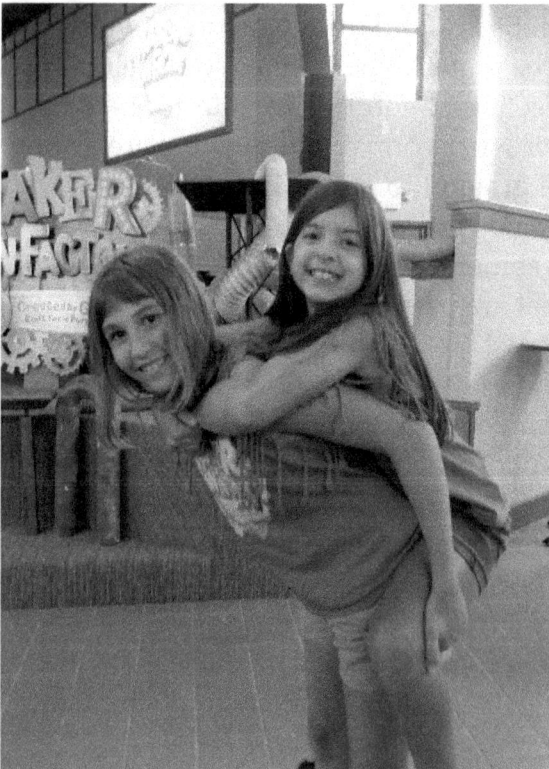

Another example might be picking up trash on the sides of roads. That would be giving back to the environment. Ask your parents if you can volunteer at your church or at a local charity. Save up money you earn and get soaps and toothpaste for a women's shelter. There are so many ways you can help others, and sometimes it's fun being creative to come up with ways to give back. One of the best ways to help others is also the easiest; just share a smile.

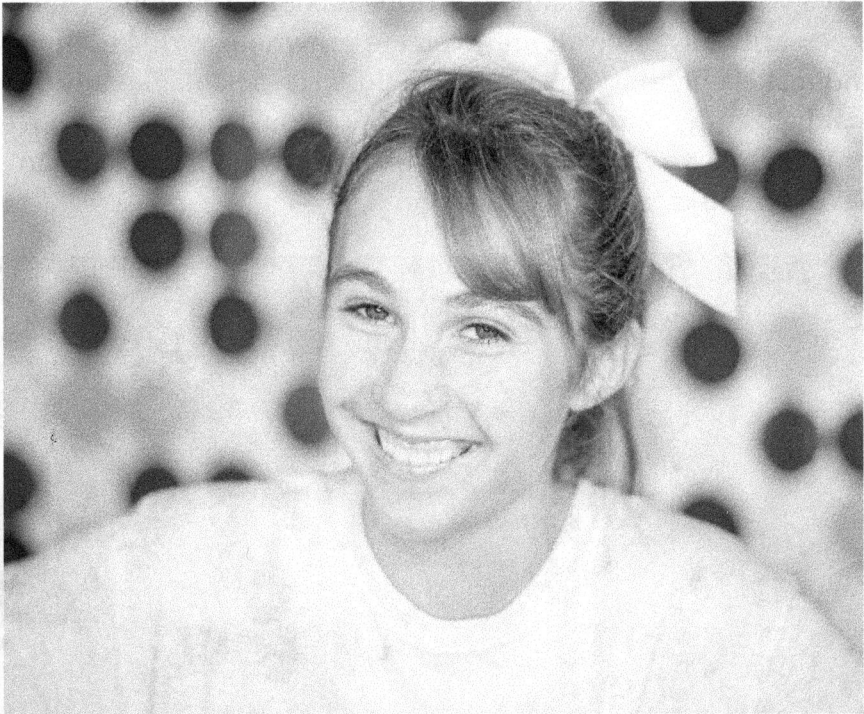

Read books

I love to read. It's always so much fun to open a book for the first time and see what adventures lurk inside. Books can help expand your vocabulary, and it's good for your mind.

A friend of mine, Caleb Maddix, actually didn't get paid to do chores when he was my age. Instead, his dad paid him for reading success books and writing a book report about them. Soon enough, he was inspired to write his own book. Then that book turned into lots of books. Now, he's still a kid and has become a successful celebrity; all from reading books, and selling his own books. That's what inspired me to write the book you're reading right now. Reading books helps your mind by teaching you things, helping with vocabulary and spelling, encouraging creativity, and helping you become more confident. The more you read, especially positive books, the more you grow.

Have you ever thought about writing a book? You don't necessarily have to wait until you are grown up to do big things and make a big difference. You could write a book like this one that helps other kids solve a problem, or you could write a novel about a fun story. Reading and writing are important skills to have ...and they are fun!

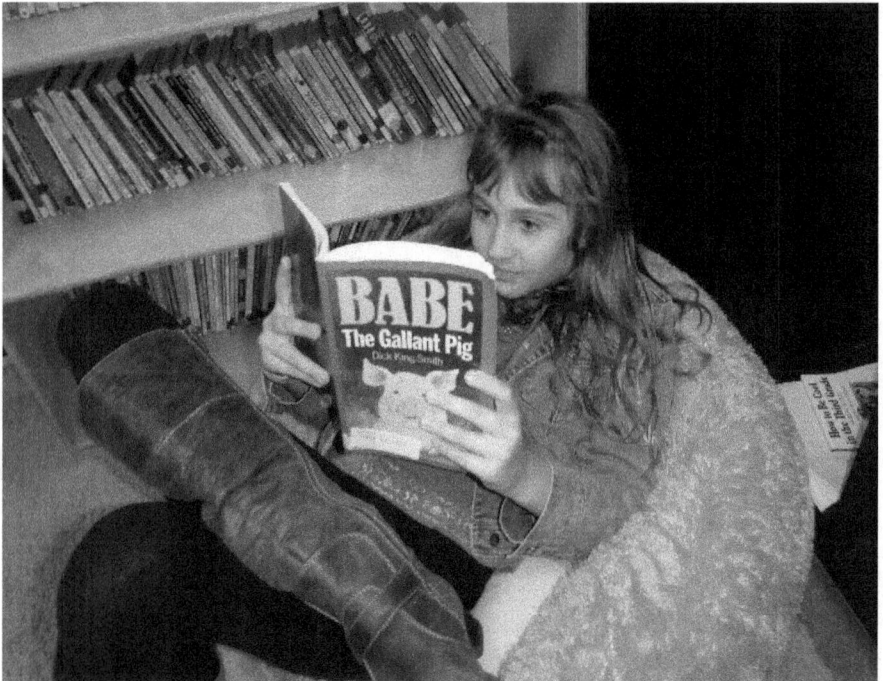

Attitude

You may have heard it said, that "Attitude is Everything." And it is so true. You are the one who controls your thoughts and feelings. Attitude, is just the reflection of what you're feeling or thinking. So, let's say your mom asks you to do the dishes. Instead of rolling your eyes and saying "Ugh. Fine!", and feeling upset doing it, you could say , "Ok!!", and just get it done. Plus you feel much better once it's over.

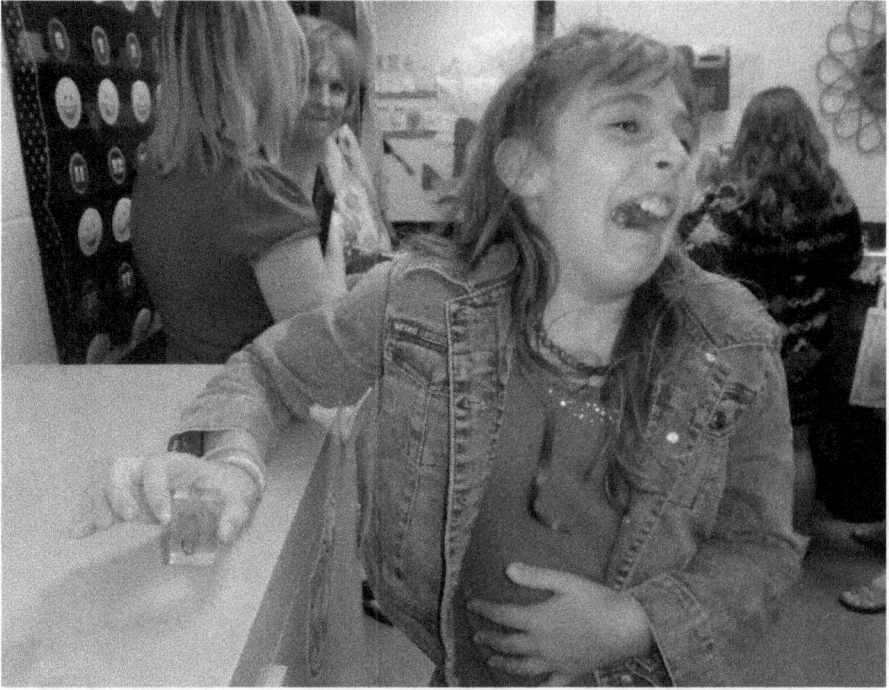

Attitude also affects outcome. I heard a quote one time that said, "What you think about, you bring about." This means, if you have a bad attitude in the morning, it can really affect your day in a negative way. And, when you have a good attitude, you tend to be more positive, nicer to others, and respond to things in a better way. As a result, you may have more friends, do better in school, have more fun, and enjoy your day.

Make sure you listen to your parents too. You may not always agree with your parents, but at least respect them. Obedience with a positive attitude can really make your parents happy, and can make you happy too.

Chapter 8
Conclusion

CONGRATULATIONS!!! YOU MADE IT THROUGH THE BOOK!!! I hope you will use the information you learned here, in your daily life. Remember what I said in the beginning of the book when I asked what you want to be when you grow up? No matter what you want to do, you need healthy habits to have success. Reading about it isn't enough, either. You have to put the healthy habits into ACTION. Remember, habits take repeating the action over and over until you don't have to think about them anymore. Now that you've read the whole book, you have an idea about some healthy habits to start with. You don't have to do them all at once. Pick one or two, make them stick, then come back and read this book again, to pick a couple more healthy habits to call your own. I believe in you and know you can do it!

Creating healthy habits is even more fun when you do it with friends. Tell your friends about this book, or better yet, give them a copy of the book.

You could even form your own "Healthy

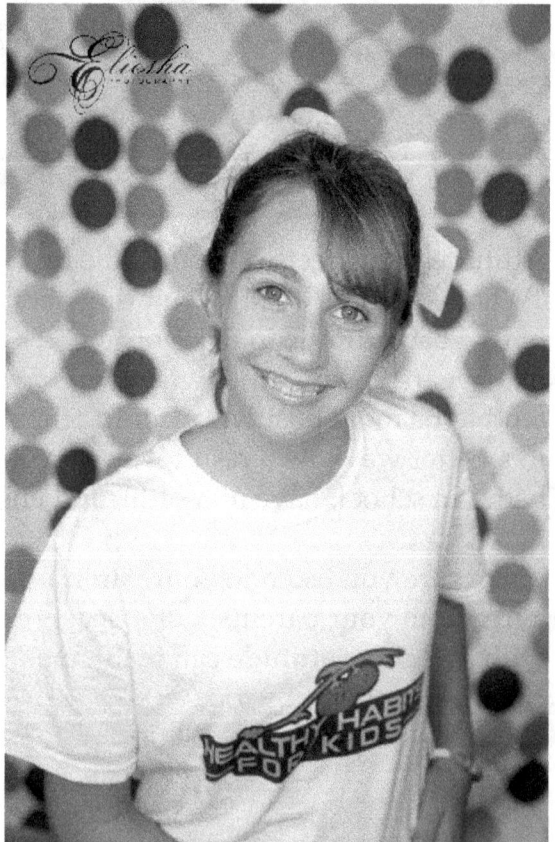

Habits for Kids" club with your friends and support each other as you learn.

Like YouTube? I sometimes help my mom make videos about healthy foods and healthy living. You can find them on our Healthy Homestead Living channel. All the videos are super kid friendly, appropriate, and clean. Even your grandma would approve.

My mom also has a website found at: www.healthyhomesteadliving.com, and she has books, tutorials, and online classes to go along with it. Why not check that out too? Anyway, I hope you learned something, take action, and create some healthy habits to last a lifetime. Farewell... for now.

God Bless,

Megan Olivia Austin

Healthy Habits

1. Eat good, healthy foods.

2. Drink lots of pure water.

3. Exercise, laugh, & have fun.

4. Keep your body, teeth, hair, and environment clean.

5. Always get enough sleep.

6. Be mentally tough, be confident, be grateful, and be positive.

7. Help others.

Chapter 9

Recipes

A fun way to enjoy healthy habits is to learn how to cook and make some of your own healthy foods. In our house, we came up with the idea that one night a week, I get to be in charge of dinner. That means I get to choose the menu and be responsible for making it. Of course, my mom helps me quite a bit including making sure we have all the ingredients needed and helping me with some of the tricky parts like using the hot oven.

Gaining skills in the kitchen is not only fun but a great way to get more confidence and independence, too. Included in the next couple pages are a few of my favorite healthier recipes for you to try. Just be careful to avoid any ingredients that you may have an allergy!

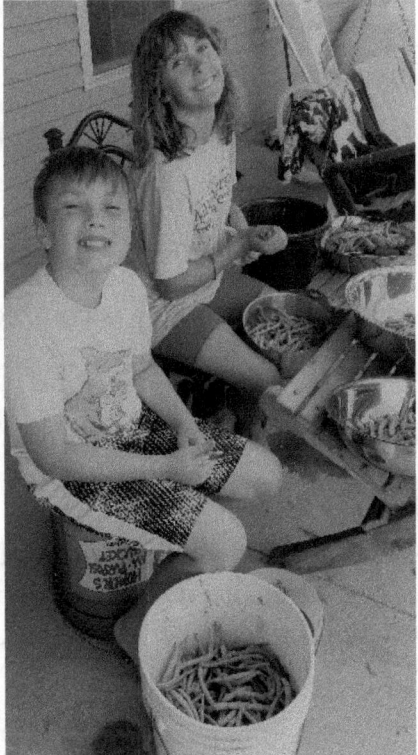

Some recipes are best done with an adult helping, especially with anything that could be dangerous like cutting with a sharp knife or using the hot stove or oven. Don't worry, though. As you practice and get better, eventually you will be able to do it all by yourself!

Homemade Lemonade

This recipe makes a super yummy and refreshing lemonade. If you want more, you can just practice some easy math and double or triple the recipe. You do need to use the stove to warm the water and dissolve the honey, so ask an adult for help if needed. There are lots of ways to get the juice out of a real lemon. One is to cut it in half and then just squeeze as hard as you can until all the juice comes out (but you'll have to dig out the seeds). Another is to use a juicer tool that helps you get the juice out by twisting ½ a cut lemon on it (but you need the tool). Careful not to accidentally squirt lemon juice in your eyes!

- *4 ½ cups purified water*

- *1/3 cup honey*

- *1 cup freshly squeezed lemon juice (from about 4-7 lemons)*

Directions:

1. Measure the water and put it in a small saucepan on the stove. Heat on low until it is warm but not boiling.

2. Remove from heat and add the honey. Stir to dissolve.

3. Once all the honey is completely dissolved, add the lemon juice and stir.

4. Taste. Add more honey if needed. Chill and enjoy!

Note: You can also add other fun ingredients like fresh mint leaves, fresh sliced strawberries, fresh raspberries, or fresh peaches for some different flavors.

Cinnamon Sunbutter

This recipe makes a really yummy alternative to peanut butter that is out of this world! Peanut butter from the store has lots of sugar and really isn't at all healthy. This version is so much better. You need a good blender or food processor to make it, though. Serve it with sliced apples for a snack or dessert.

- *1 cup sunflower seed kernels (dry, roasted, no salt)*
- *2 tablespoons olive oil*
- *1/3 cup honey*
- *Dash of salt (remember, Celtic or Himalayan is best)*
- *½ tsp cinnamon*

Directions:

1. Combine all ingredients in a food processor and pulse until creamy.

2. Serve with sliced apples.

Note: You can also add 4 ounces of cream cheese for a variation that is super good.

Chocolate Hummus Dip

Personally I don't love hummus even though I know it has lots of healthy ingredients. I do enjoy chocolate, though, and this dip is great for snacking or even dessert. Use it with apple slices, strawberries, blueberries, crackers, or add it to a sandwich. You'll need a food processor, which makes this recipe super easy to make. This recipe uses an ingredient called cacao powder which is the superfood version of cocoa powder. Mom says it has lots of nutrients like magnesium.

- *2 cups canned chickpeas (garbanzo beans)*

- *4 tablespoons cacao powder*

- *2 tablespoons almond butter*

- *¼ cup pure maple syrup*

- *1 teaspoon vanilla*

Directions:

1. Add all ingredients to a food processor and pulse/ puree until smooth.

2. Serve or chill for later use.

Frozen Yogurt Pops

I love popsicles and frozen sweet treats. Too often, though, the ones we get at the store have too much sugar. Making your own is fun and easy… and the best part is that you can get really creative on the flavors you make! Use your imagination and feel free to experiment to find your favorites. You can use paper muffin cups to make these. We use the silicone muffin cups, though, and they pop right out after freezing with no mess (and they're reusable for less waste).

- *1 cup plain, unsweetened yogurt*

- *1 medium banana*

- *1 cup frozen fruit of choice (mixed berries, peach, strawberry, blueberry, mango, kiwi, blackberry, etc.)*

- *1/8 cup honey*

- *Popsicle sticks*

Directions:

1. Place all ingredients into a high-powered blender and puree until smooth.

2. Place paper or silicone muffin cups into a muffin tin. Mini muffin tins are great too for mini- popsicles.

3. Divide yogurt mixture evenly between the cups.

4. Place in the freezer (keep them level) for 1 hour.

5. Remove and insert popsicle sticks in the center of each pop.

6. Put them back in the freezer until completely frozen.

7. Enjoy!

Kale Chips

Who says eating greens can't be tasty? I was actually surprised how good these were the first time I had them. Once you start eating them, it'll be hard to stop! Kale is easy to grow yourself, too. If you have space for a garden where you live, you might ask about growing your own. Get some help from an adult on these for the oven part of the recipe, just to be safe.

- *4 cups kale leaves, washed*

- *2 tablespoons coconut oil*

- *Juice from ½ medium lemon*

- *¼ teaspoon Celtic or Himalayan sea salt*

Directions:

1. Preheat oven to 375° F. Prepare a baking sheet with parchment paper.

2. Chop or tear by hand, about 4 cups of kale leaves, removing the tough middle stem.

3. Place all the ingredients in a large bowl.

4. This is where it gets fun! Massage the kale leaves with your hands, mixing in all the other ingredients at the same time. Massaging the kale makes it tender and will coat the leaves with the salt, oil, and lemon.

5. Place on a parchment-paper lined baking sheet.

6. Bake for 12 minutes until crispy but not burned.

Homemade French Fries

Once you taste your own homemade fries and see how easy they are to make, you'll never want drive-through again. Well, maybe, but still they're so much better. AND, they are much healthier, too. Be sure to ask an adult for help with the oven and cutting if needed.

- *3-4 large baking potatoes*

- *1 tablespoon coconut oil, melted*

- *1 teaspoon Celtic or Himalayan sea salt*

Directions:

1. Preheat oven to 425° F and prepare a baking sheet by lining it with parchment paper.

2. Wash potatoes and cut them carefully into 3/8- inch strips. You can leave the skins on.

3. Place potatoes and oil in a plastic bag and shake until the potatoes are coated in oil.

4. Arrange in a single layer on the baking sheet.

5. Bake for 15 minutes. Have an adult help you turn the potatoes over, sprinkle lightly with salt, and bake another 5 minutes or until done to your desired crispness.

Pancakes

Seriously, pancakes are one of my favorite foods. I could eat them any time of day! And, if you use the right ingredients, they can be quite healthy, too! Made from scratch and using pure, maple syrup avoids all the unhealthy stuff found in store-bought mixes and syrups. And, they taste so much better!

- *2 eggs*
- *2 cups buttermilk or almond milk*
- *2 teaspoons vanilla*
- *1 ¾ cups Einkorn flour (or you can use spelt, kamut, or almond flour)*
- *2 teaspoons baking powder*
- *1 teaspoon baking soda*
- *½ teaspoon Celtic or Himalayan salt*

Directions:

1. With adult help, heat griddle or large skillet over medium heat.

2. In a large bowl, add the eggs, being careful not to get any shells. Stir in the milk and vanilla.

3. Add the remaining ingredients and mix until most of the lumps disappear.

4. Lightly grease the griddle with some butter. Carefully drop about ¼ cup of batter onto the griddle. Let cook about 2 minutes or until bubbles form.

5. Carefully flip pancake and cook other side for another 30 seconds or so until done.

6. Repeat process with remaining batter.

7. Serve warm with butter and maple syrup.

Homemade Chicken Nuggets

I know I said earlier that processed chicken nuggets weren't very healthy, but these are delicious and good for you too! They're fun to make because you get to use your fingers in the batter. Just ask an adult to help with the oven, to be safe. Note, leave out the nuts if you are allergic.

- *¼ cup Einkorn flour (or you can use almond flour, spelt, or kamut)*

- *½ teaspoon seasoned salt*

- *1 cup finely chopped pecans or almonds*

- *4 boneless, skinless, organic chicken breast halves, cut into 1 inch pieces*

- *¼ cup melted butter*

Directions:

1. Preheat oven to 400° F.

2. In a plastic ziplock-style bag, combine chicken, flour, and salt.

3. Shake the bag to mix (But be careful not to break open the bag. This makes a big mess. I know!)

4. Dip floured pieces of chicken into the melted butter to coat and then roll in the crushed nuts until evenly covered.

5. Place on a baking sheet and bake for 15-20 minutes, or until the chicken is fully cooked (no pink when you cut it open).

Chocolate Chip Cookies

My mom came up with this recipe when my dad was recovering from cancer and we couldn't have any sugar or grains. I love these cookies, and like them just as much as the original. They have a more cake-like texture than regular cookies with that melt-in-your mouth flavor.

- *2 cups Almond Flour*
- *½ cup softened (not melted) Butter or coconut oil*
- *¼ to 1/3 cup "Cup-for-Cup" Stevia*
- *1 large egg*
- *½ teaspoons Baking Soda*
- *pinch of Celtic Salt*
- *1 tablespoon pure Vanilla*
- *1 cup (or less) Lily's Stevia Sweetened Chocolate Chips*

Directions:

1. Preheat oven to 350° F.

2. Mix the almond flour, baking soda, stevia, and salt in a bowl. Add the softened butter or coconut oil (or a mix of both) and stir well by hand until mixed. It should form a thick dough that is hard to stir.

3. Add the egg and mix well. This should make the dough more formable and easier to mix. If needed, add a tsp or two of milk to thin. Finished dough should be easy to form.

4. Add chocolate chips and stir by hand until incorporated.

5. Form dough into tablespoon size balls and bake for 10 minutes or until tops are starting to be golden brown.

6. Let cool at least 5 minutes and serve.